The Overeater's Journal

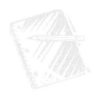

Exercises for the Heart, Mind, and Soul

Debbie Danowski, Ph.D.

HAZELDEN

Hazelden
Center City, Minnesota 55012-0176

1-800-328-0094
1-651-213-4590 (Fax)
www.hazelden.org

ISBN: 978-1-59285-080-8

12 11 10 09   6 5 4 3

Interior design by Rachel Holscher
Typesetting by Stanton Publication Services, Inc.

This book is dedicated to Melissa for giving me hope during my darkest hours and for always making me feel special.

Contents

Acknowledgments

This past year I faced perhaps the greatest challenge I have ever known in recovery—a divorce. In a heartbreaking twist of fate, my soul mate and I were unable to make our relationship work. After almost twelve years together, we made the decision to end our marriage. Perhaps the single saddest day in my life was when the judge declared our marriage to be dissolved.

Though legally it was relatively simple to end our marriage, emotionally it has been a devastating experience to be out of touch with the person who was my best friend for most of my recovering life. And though we are not together, I could not write this section without acknowledging the role that my former husband has played in my writing career. It was with his love and support that I was able to publish my first two books that served as the basis for this one and for that I will be forever grateful.

Similarly, both this book and my recovery would not be possible without the love and support of so many wonderful people in my life. To begin, my parents, Ann and Andy, have served as the guiding force in my life. I know that without their love and support I could not have made it through not only the past year, but also my entire life. They have been there for me whenever I have needed them, and there are no words to express how much that means to me.

No less important are my siblings. My sister, Karen, her husband, Danny, and my niece, Melissa, have all been an important part of both my life and my recovery. I cannot count the number of times that all of them have gone out of their way to make sure I made it through the past year. And Melissa continues to be the light in my life that carries me through my darkest moments just by being herself. My life is so much richer because of her presence.

My brother, Mike, and his wife, Denise, have been an amazing support to me throughout this experience as well. I cannot express how much strength I gain from knowing that they are in my life. My extended family has also served as a source of support and provided me with hope throughout the entire writing process.

Similarly, my friends have served as an incredible support system for me both during the past year and throughout my life. And though each and every one of them has a special place in my heart, it is difficult to put into words how much Bev Robillard has touched my life with the support and friendship that she so freely provides. Other friends who have shared their love and support with me are Rich Mayo, Paulette Day, Mark Egmon, Jennie Hendrix, and Chris O'Hearn.

As a writer, it is necessary to develop a support group of people who provide motivation when no one else seems to. For me, Dawn Rosner, Mark Edwards, Amanda Veautour, Jane Pollak, and Dr. Mike Ventimiglia have encouraged my writing and listened to me regularly. For this, I am extremely grateful.

As a recovering person, my network of support people is an incredible gift in my life. I could not have made it through one minute of abstinence if it were not for the love and support of so many people who are walking the road to recovery with me. My heartfelt thanks go to Roger, Alex, Linda, Elaine, Vickie, Kim, Adria, Jill, Joan, Ruth, Jocelyn, Frank, and everyone else who shares my disease. No less important is my online support group that motivates me even when I am exhausted. Thanks to Josie, Wendy, Tina, Cara, Rita, Rachel, Tracy, Leonora, Joan, Robyn, Jess, Ann, and everyone else who takes the time to post a message at the most supportive place on the Internet.

The struggle to live a healthy lifestyle is often challenging, but some people have made it easier. I am grateful to Jack de Graffenried for being a wonderful and supportive workout partner, who pushes me to do more than I ever thought I could. I am also grateful to have found a gym where I feel comfortable enough to exercise in front of other people. It is a credit to those at World Gym in Trumbull that the environment there is loving and supportive.

I am also very grateful for the children in my life who remind me that fun is an important part of recovery. From the day she was born Melissa has continually taught me how to play and have fun, often leading me to playgrounds, amusement parks, and bowling alleys. And from Felicia Stolz and JJ de Graffenried, I have learned to be fearless and enthusiastic in my play. I am truly grateful for every moment that I spend with each one.

Professionally, there are too many people who have helped me along the way to name all of them, but I will do my best. At Sacred Heart, I am grateful to be blessed with wonderful, caring co-workers on every level, but especially in both the English and media studies departments, including Beverly Boehmke, Dr. Jeff Cain,

Dr. Bunny Calabrese, Dr. Jim Castonguay, Dr. Ralph Corrigan, Dr. David Curtis, Dr. Angela DiPace, Carol Esposito, Greg Golda, Dr. Sid Gottlieb, Dr. Michelle Loris, Dr. Rick Magee, Dr. Robin McAllister, Dr. Andy Miller, Dr. Judy Miller, Dr. Louise Spence, Dr. Roberta Staples, Dr. Sylvia Watts, and Dr. Sandy Young.

Just as wonderful are the people at Hazelden who believed in me from the beginning. As my first editor, Corrine Casanova will always hold a special place in my life. I am also grateful to my current editor, Karen Chernyaev, for her support and encouragement in writing this book. All of those at Hazelden who have touched my life have helped to make me a better writer. Thanks, too, to Joan Flavell for the cover design and Monica Dwyer Abress for her copyediting.

Finally, I offer my sincerest gratitude to God for the life and work He has given me.

Introduction

The title of this book contains the word *overeater*, and the phrase *food addict* is used throughout the journal. However, it's important to note that the exercises in this journal can be used by those who regularly gain and lose the same fifteen pounds, those who are underweight, and even those who are at a healthy weight but have an unhealthy relationship with food. A food addict is physically and emotionally dependent on certain food substances, such as sugar, flour, fat, and sometimes wheat, to the point that these substances interfere with normal daily functioning.

Although *food addict* may seem like a contradiction in terms (we all need to eat after all), it refers to the compulsive need to overeat when triggered by certain substances or emotions. Nonaddicted people oftentimes have similar attitudes and behaviors that create an unhealthy relationship with food. Therefore, the continued use of the term *food addict* is done for ease of writing but may be translated to include all of the previously mentioned groups. Some of the entries in this journal may seem intense, but they can assist anyone who is unhappy with his or her relationship with food.

This journal provides you with simple yet thought-provoking writing exercises that will aid your food addiction recovery. Although it may be difficult at first to make the connection between writing and food addiction recovery, it's not as difficult as you may think. Many professionals have regularly linked writing with healing. For example, M. White and D. Epston argue that the "written tradition" should be used regularly in therapy. They point out that it "provides for an expansion of the information that can be processed in our short-term memory at any one point in time."[1] Similarly, describing a patient who had used letter writing to confront sexual abuse, T. Vance points out the following:

> And although she had talked in therapy about the abuse she suffered growing up, she had never gone into such detail. Writing helped her integrate her trauma in a way that gave her perspective. For the first time, she could talk about the experiences and feelings without reexperiencing shame and guilt.[2]

Furthermore, in a study by E. F. Nye where AIDS patients were asked to write weekly journal entries, the conclusion was that writing served as a means of healing.[3]

The disease of food addiction is a threefold affliction—physical, emotional, and spiritual—and the journal writing exercises in this book reflect each of these areas. Because it is generally believed that emotional and spiritual recovery are more difficult until the physical aspect of the disease is addressed, the physical section comes first. In this section, you will examine your food intake, eating patterns, and beliefs. The section that addresses the emotional aspects of food addiction will help you to discover those feelings that you associate with overeating. In the final section, you will be guided through exercises that allow you to examine your spiritual beliefs as related to recovery and life.

As with all journal writing exercises, the single most important element is honesty. You are writing this journal for you and no one else. It is not going to be graded or judged or critiqued. You are simply writing to help you recover from your food addiction. The only person who ever has to read this, unless you choose otherwise, is you. There is no audience here, and you are not writing to please anyone. Your writing is your own personal business. And even though it may be difficult at first, it's important to remember that the greater your honesty, the more solid your recovery will eventually be.

Sometimes it is helpful to think of your journal as a friend who will never judge you or reveal your secrets. Think how it would feel to share your deepest secrets with someone who will never say a harsh word or criticize you. Even more, consider what a wonderful feeling it would be to have total acceptance of what you consider to be your most blatant and troublesome character flaws. All of this is possible within the pages of this book. The only thing you have to do to enjoy all of these benefits is to write.

It's vital that you be aware of the resistance you may face when writing in this journal. In most cases, you will be your biggest obstacle. From the time that you first began using food as more than a means of nourishing your body, your addictive thinking did whatever it took to protect you from being aware of how dangerous your actions were. Throughout your overeating history, a part of you has been in denial about your behavior. Before you go judging yourself, realize that denial is a hallmark of any addiction and that you are not the first or only person to ever do this.

The important point is that you take steps to overcome this denial. The journal exercises are designed to assist you, but realize that your mind will resist your efforts to be totally honest. Try to think of having two voices in your head. One voice is healthy and wants to break through the denial and be in recovery. The other voice is that of your disease. This voice wants you to continue overeating and works hard at keeping you out of recovery. It is this voice that will speak loudest to you when you begin writing. Sometimes it will be obvious, telling you that you don't need to write or questioning whether writing will actually help. Other times, however, it will be very subtle, suggesting that you do something more important than writing or that you are being selfish for taking time out of your day to write. The voice of addiction does not want to lose its power and will do what it can to keep you actively addicted to overeating.

While you can't make these voices disappear, eventually they will wane, and with discipline they will diminish. This is not to suggest that you fight these voices but rather acknowledge their presence and write anyway. One of the most effective ways of breaking through denial and working toward recovery is to write on a regular basis at around the same time each day. In other words, if you set aside fifteen minutes each day at the same time, writing will become a habit just like brushing your teeth or showering. By making writing a habit, you will take away any internal debate you may be having with yourself.

Still not convinced? Take into consideration the words of others who have used writing to help in their recoveries. First, a woman who struggled with weight loss for thirty years discovered the benefits of journal writing when dealing with behavior changes.

My previous diet attempts have always been thwarted by some emotionally traumatic event. It may have been as minor as a broken fingernail or as major as the death of my mother, but always with the same result— I would lose my momentum and eventually drift away from the whole diet.

In one last attempt, this morbidly obese woman at 235 pounds decided to try keeping a daily journal to aid her in dealing with her feelings.

> Not a "diet diary," not a journal of my weight-loss progress or eating problems, but a journal to keep me emotionally on track. I simply write about what is happening in my life, good or bad. I write out my anger, my frustrations, my unhappiness. Before, when I felt miserable, I'd eat and cry and stare out the window wondering why I felt that way. Writing helps me to get my problems off my mind and onto paper, so I don't feel the compulsion to eat.[4]

A recovering member of Overeaters Anonymous has used writing to assist in the process of inventorying those personality traits causing her difficulties in recovery. She says the following:

> I took out my notebook and wrote, even though it wasn't what I thought I should write; no past history or list of defects, simply what was causing me anxiety at the moment. The next day I reread what I'd written and began again, this time putting down similar feelings and behaviors from the past. I was encouraged and enthused as I glimpsed the benefits of inventory writing.
>
> Quick thinking may be great in its place, but it is a handicap when it comes to in-depth inventory taking. Writing slows down my thought processes and enables me to backtrack over the thoughts I have expressed on paper. This increases my self-awareness far beyond what was possible over the kitchen sink. As I wrote, I could see threads weaving through my life, all connected to certain key defects. These defects were causing me a great deal of pain.[5]

The Overeaters Anonymous member describes perhaps the most important element in food addiction recovery: the ability to increase self-awareness. <u>Self-awareness is the most powerful weapon in the battle against a strong denial mechanism that constantly hides the true dangers of food addiction from its victims.</u>

Now, it's your turn. You've done enough reading about the benefits of journal writing and the way in which this book is organized. The time has come for you to pick up your pen and write.

And just in case you are thinking of ways to get around it, consider the words of well-known journal expert Ira Progoff:

> Thinking about what you would write is not the same as actually writing it. The act of writing in the atmosphere that is created by the journal process at work and that builds cumulatively as you follow the format of its exercises seems to evoke depths in us that mere thinking does not reach. . . . You will find that the act of . . . actually recording [your thoughts] in written form has the effect of stimulating a movement within you that draws forth awareness you would not have thought of in advance.[6]

The awareness that Progoff mentions is vital for food addiction recovery. Without a deep-level awareness of the dangers involved in food addiction, its victims remain unable or unwilling to take action and move toward recovery.

How can I be so sure? Well, if you read *Locked Up for Eating Too Much,* you know that journal writing saved my life. As a 328-pound woman, I was on my way to an early death when I entered a treatment center in Tampa, Florida. During my six-week stay there, I was required to keep a daily journal. And even though I didn't like writing every day, as time went on, I began to discover aspects of my personality that I never even imagined to be true.

In the pages of my journal, I was free to explore my deepest, most humiliating experiences with food and eating. Most of these were insights that I had never even thought about until I wrote them down. Somehow the act of writing forced me to make sense of what I had kept hidden for so long. And by uncovering these things, I was able to deal with them and acknowledge my food addiction. This acknowledgment eventually led to a 175-pound weight loss and an entirely new way of life.

As part of my new way of life, I have made it my mission to help others who suffer from food addiction. To that end, I have published two books to help other food addicts. *Why Can't I Stop Eating?* with coauthor Pedro Lazaro, M.D., outlines a program of recovery for those addicted to food. The second book, *Locked Up for*

Eating Too Much, describes my experiences in a food addiction treatment center, which includes my journals from the treatment center. It is within those pages that a hopelessly disillusioned girl wrote her way into a recovery that has lasted fourteen years and resulted in a better life than she ever dreamed possible.

So now it's up to you. When making your final decision about whether to actually do the exercises in this book, think about S. W. Albert's beliefs. "Written words are stronger, surer. They have a longer lease-hold, a greater half-life. Because they are more substantial, they demand more in the making and offer more potential for the long term."[7] This being so, the exercises in this book may offer you benefits you never even dreamed of. So turn the page and begin writing. Your life may depend on it!

I'd love to hear about your journal writing experiences. Feel free to contact me by e-mail at danowskid@sacredheart.edu or by postal mail at Debbie Danowski, 4 Daniels Farm Road #193, Trumbull, CT 06611. You can also post a message at my Web site at www.debbiedanowski.com.

The Overeater's Journal

Section One

Physical

What Did I Eat Today?

Failing to plan is planning to fail.

Unknown

For a food addict, writing out a daily food plan is an important part of recovery. Making food choices throughout the day without planning is dangerous. Without a plan, someone who has been conditioned through years of practice to use food for other reasons rather than eating will reach for something unhealthy. So where do you begin? Start by making a plan in the morning or the night before to provide you with the insurance you need against bingeing and relapse.

On the following page you will find a food log. Make copies of this page so that you can use it daily. Not only will this exercise help you to better plan your meals, but it will also allow you to chart your progress.

At the end of the exercise, you will find an area where you can write about your feelings regarding your food choices for the day. The most important element in this area is honesty. Over the years, most food addicts have made it a habit to lie about what they eat. Overcoming this tendency is the single most important step in recovery. No matter how painful it may seem at first, be honest about both your food choices and the feelings surrounding them.

	What I planned to eat:	What I ate:
Breakfast:	_____	_____
	_____	_____
Lunch:	_____	_____
	_____	_____
Dinner:	_____	_____
	_____	_____
Snack(s):	_____	_____
	_____	_____

How do I feel about my food choices today?

_____

_____

What, if anything, would I change?

_____

_____

If I plan to change things, what action can I take immediately to begin?

_____

_____

Am I Dishonest?

A liar needs a good memory.

Quintilian

One of the most obvious signs of food addiction is dishonesty. Ashamed by excessive eating behavior, most food addicts lie about the amount and types of food they've eaten. The pattern of lying becomes so ingrained in a food addict's makeup that he or she is oftentimes unable to discern the truth.

A big part of recovery is being honest about both past and present behaviors. Though it may not be easy, it is important for you to be as honest as you possibly can when answering the following questions. Remember, you don't have to show this to anyone else, but if you truly want to live a healthy and happy life, you will need to become honest about your eating patterns.

How often do you lie about the amount and/or types of foods you have eaten? Name at least three recent specific incidents.

_____

_____

_____

_____

_____

_____

After you have been untruthful how do you feel?

_____

_____

_____

Name four reasons why you lie and discuss what you think would happen if you were truthful.

_____

_____

_____

_____

_____

_____

_____

If you were to be honest about your eating, whom would you choose to tell? What do you think his or her reaction would be?

_____

_____

_____

What would it feel like to be completely honest about what you have eaten?

_____

_____

_____

How Much of My Time Involves Food?

Destiny is not a matter of chance, it is a matter of choice,
it is not a thing to be waited for, but something
to be achieved.

William Jennings Bryan

Food addicts live with the mistaken belief that things just happen to them without any action or say on their part. One of the most difficult things a food addict has to realize is that his or her actions directly affect the quality of life he or she lives.

Keep a log of the amount of time you spend shopping for, preparing, eating, and thinking about food. Do not try to do this from memory. Instead write down the events as soon as possible after they occur. Though you can do this for one day, it would be better to keep a log for at least two days if not more.

Shopping: If you stopped at a food store or went to a restaurant or fast-food place, record it below. Be sure to include travel time.

Time began   Time ended   Total

_____

_____

_____

_____

Preparing: Make a list of the amount of time you spent preparing food. Be sure to include time spent washing, cutting up, peeling, mixing, measuring, etc.

Time began   Time ended   Total

_____

_____

_____

_____

Eating: Write down the amount of time you spent eating. Remember to include even small snacks or any time you put food into your mouth, not just full meals.

Time began   Time ended   Total

_____

_____

_____

_____

Thinking about Food: Each and every occasion food comes into your mind, write it down. Be sure to include any time spent looking at recipes, cookbooks, or talking about food.

Time began   Time ended   Total

_____

_____

_____

_____

What Else Can I Do Instead of Eating?

The undertaking of a new action brings new strength.

Evenius

Even though it may seem impossible right now to stop spending so much of your time with food, realize that there is another way of life. There are other things that you can spend your time on that will give you a lot more satisfaction. Keep in mind that by trying new things, you will become even stronger.

To begin, look at the previous exercise and add up the amount of time in the "Total" column of each section. When you have a number for each section, add these together for a final total of the amount of your time that involves food. Then use this figure to answer the following questions. Remember, even if you don't like the answers you are coming up with, it's important to be honest. By writing all of this information down, you are helping yourself to move closer to recovery. Isn't that worth it?

How much of your day revolves around food?

1. Time spent awake (24 hours minus time spent sleeping): _____ hrs.

2. Total time spent with food (from log on pp. 8–9): _____ hrs.

3. Total time spent WITHOUT food: _____ hrs.

What, if anything, surprised you about these numbers? Do you have any concerns? If so, write about them.

_____

_____

_____

_____

When looking at the different times that you entered, what conclusions can you make about how you spend time with food? Does thinking about food take up most of your day? Or do you spend the majority of your time preparing and eating food?

_____

_____

_____

_____

Write down four things (not necessarily food related) that you have always wanted to do but never could find the time. How long would it take to do each of these things?

_____

_____

_____

_____

_____

_____

_____

What Are My Binge Foods?

Admitting error clears the score—
and proves you wiser than before.

Arthur Guiterman

As you already know, one of the most difficult aspects of recovery is being honest about overeating. Now that you've completed some journaling exercises to help with being truthful, it's time to discover your binge foods. Before you begin, it's important to realize that your first instinct will be to deny that some of your biggest binge foods are actually causing problems. To help overcome this powerful denial mechanism, write down as much as possible. In other words, if you're in doubt, write it down anyway. If you need more space, go on to another sheet of paper, but whatever you do, don't stop writing until you've gotten it all out.

Make a list of those foods you eat on a regular basis. If you need to, refer to the food log on page 5.

_____

_____

_____

From the list above, write down those foods that you regularly overeat.

_____

_____

_____

Now list foods about which you think and/or fantasize. (You may not necessarily eat these foods regularly.)

_____

_____

_____

What foods do you think you couldn't possibly live without? Why?

_____

_____

_____

Write down those foods that have special meaning in your life. Think about those foods you use to celebrate special events or holidays, you use to console yourself, or you cook for others.

_____

_____

_____

Write down the foods that appear on at least two of these lists.

_____

_____

_____

The foods written above are your binge foods. How does this feel?

_____

_____

_____

What Substances Am I Using?

Nature has given us the seeds of knowledge,
not knowledge itself.

Lucius Seneca

It's time to determine what substances are present in your binge foods. Once again, honesty is crucial. Try to think of this exercise as a scavenger hunt rather than a condemnation of your eating habits. To thoroughly complete this exercise, you will need to read the labels on some of the foods you have eaten. It is not necessary, however, to buy or have these foods in your home. Having these foods readily available is dangerous to your recovery and certainly not necessary for your journal writing. One trip to the grocery store should allow you to gather all the information you will need. Ask a friend to help if a trip to the store is too full of temptation.

Take a look at the items listed in the previous exercise as your binge foods. Now write down the first five ingredients listed on the labels of each.

_____ _____ _____ _____ _____

_____ _____ _____ _____ _____

_____ _____ _____ _____ _____

_____ _____ _____ _____ _____

_____ _____ _____ _____ _____

Next, make a list of those items that appear most frequently.

_____

_____

Put a check by the ingredients in the following list that are in your binge foods.

❏ barley malt   ❏ honey   ❏ brown sugar
❏ invert sugar   ❏ cane sugar   ❏ lactose
❏ corn sweetener   ❏ maltose   ❏ corn syrup
❏ mannitol   ❏ dextrose   ❏ maple syrup
❏ fructose   ❏ sorghum   ❏ glucose
❏ sorbitol   ❏ grape sugar   ❏ sucrose
❏ grape sweetener   ❏ high fructose corn syrup

All of these ingredients are different forms of sugar. How do you feel about the number of check marks you made?

_____

_____

Looking at the following list, put a check by those ingredients that are in your binge foods.

❏ flour   ❏ wheat flour   ❏ rye flour
❏ corn flour   ❏ rice flour   ❏ corn meal

What is the primary ingredient(s) in most of your binge foods? Why do you think this is?

_____

_____

Do you feel you are physically addicted to certain food substances?

_____

_____

What Does It Mean to Be Addicted?

Do what you can, with what you have, where you are.

Theodore Roosevelt

When many of us think about the word *addiction,* images of drug-addicted junkies may come to mind. Though this may be the case sometimes, it is not the whole picture. An addict can be the person who gambles or drinks too much or even the one who shops or uses sex to the extreme. While you may have heard of people having these addictions, the idea of being addicted to food may still seem unbelievable to you. Before you make any final judgments about this concept or your own life, complete this exercise.

Someone with an addiction is driven to use his or her substance. Do you feel it is this way with food for you? Why or why not?

_____

_____

_____

_____

_____

What does the word *addiction* mean to you? Do you feel that you are addicted to food? Why or why not?

_____

_____

_____

_____

_____

According to the book *Alcoholics Anonymous,* the craving an addict experiences is "beyond all mental control."[8] How does this relate to the various weight-loss methods you have tried?

_____

_____

_____

_____

_____

Discuss in detail the number of weight-loss methods you have tried.

_____

_____

_____

_____

_____

What Consequences Do I Have from Overeating?

Erasmus must feed himself and wear his own feathers.

Erasmus

With an addiction, there are many consequences. For people addicted to alcohol or other drugs, this may mean deteriorated health, legal difficulties, financial ramifications, or even broken relationships. Though food addicts may experience many of these same things, there tends to be a reluctance or inability to equate these consequences with overeating. Though it may not seem important, realizing the consequences of your addiction is a vital step on the road to recovery. When writing, try not to judge yourself. Just simply write.

Physical consequences are common with food addiction. Write about yours. Think about your body size, your health, and your ability to move around.

_____

_____

_____

_____

_____

What activities has your body size and/or lack of energy prevented you from participating in?

_____

_____

_____

_____

Write about the role your addiction has played in your relationships.

_____

_____

_____

Financially, how much money have you spent on your addiction? Remember to include not only food but weight-loss programs, clothes, cookbooks, cooking utensils and appliances, antacids, painkillers, and health care.

_____

_____

_____

_____

After looking at the previous questions, how severe do you feel the consequences of your addiction have been? What are your feelings about this?

_____

_____

_____

_____

Have I Hit Bottom?

The hardest thing to learn in life is which bridge to
cross and which to burn.

David Russell

For many food addicts, hitting bottom means the beginning of making life changes. Addicts become willing to do anything to take the necessary steps toward a new life. In this journal exercise, you will be asked to determine whether or not you have reached this point of willingness. While it isn't always necessary to experience an intense amount of pain to recover, you will need to be motivated to make changes. It's up to you to decide what motivates you.

Make a list of all of the foods you've overeaten. Include as many as you possibly can. For help, refer to the binge list you created on page 13.

_____

_____

_____

_____

_____

Now write about the amount of food you've overeaten. For instance, did you eat one half-gallon of ice cream or two? Whatever it is, write it down.

_____

_____

_____

_____

_____

Take some time to find a suggested healthy eating plan. You can use the governmental recommendations (USDA Food Pyramid) as a guideline. For more detailed information on writing a personalized food plan, consult my book *Why Can't I Stop Eating?* There is a whole chapter devoted to this topic.

What does hitting bottom mean to you? Do you feel you have hit your bottom? Why or why not?

_____

_____

_____

_____

_____

When looking for a healthy eating plan, do not use traditional diet plans as the majority of those programs include foods that are dangerous to food addicts.

What's the Worst Binge I Ever Had?

A problem well stated is a problem half solved.

Charles F. Kettering

Knowing exactly how serious your overeating behavior has become is vital to making changes and moving toward recovery. Though it may not be pleasant to write about the worst binge you've ever had, it is necessary to learn how severe the problem is. Being aware of the seriousness of the situation allows you the foundation to begin solving the problem. Remember, you control the ownership of this journal and no one else will see your words. Be honest in your answers.

Recalling as many details as you can, write down what you ate during the worst binge you've ever had. Be specific about the types and amounts of food as well as the time period over which this binge took place.

_____

_____

_____

_____

_____

_____

Make a list of the foods you ate in this binge in the order in which you ate them.

_____

_____

_____

_____

Beginning with the first food item and working your way through to the last, write what your feelings were before you ate each food item. If you are unsure, choose from the following four basic feelings: glad, mad, sad, scared. Be as specific as possible.

_____

_____

_____

_____

Working through the list again, write what your feelings were while you were eating and after you were finished.

_____

_____

_____

Take a minute to review the lists you've made in this exercise. How serious do you think your overeating is? Explain.

_____

_____

_____

Do I Know What Physical Cravings Are?

These men were not drinking to escape; they were
drinking to overcome a craving beyond their mental
control. . . . They cannot start drinking without
developing the phenomenon of craving.

William D. Silkworth, M.D.

Following is an excerpt from *Why Can't I Stop Eating?* describing physical cravings:

One of the most important facts we have learned about food over the
years is that certain foods react negatively in a person's system, which
causes the person to overeat. As soon as these substances enter the system, a person physically craves more and more of them, and no matter
how much is eaten, it will never be enough. Just as an alcoholic physically craves alcohol, some people physically crave certain foods. . . .

It is this physical craving for substances that causes individuals to
overeat. In the same manner that, after years of drinking, alcoholics become dependent on alcohol, food addicts desire food.[9]

How does the information in the excerpt on page 24 manifest itself in your life?

_____

_____

_____

_____

_____

_____

Do you believe you have experienced the "phenomenon of craving" beyond your "mental control" that Dr. Silkworth describes? If so, write about both a specific incident and throughout your life.

_____

_____

_____

_____

_____

_____

_____

Do I Know What a Normal Portion Is?

I can give you a six-word formula for success:
Think things through—then follow through.

Eddie Rickenbacker

Part of recovering from food addiction and learning to manage your overeating is thinking in new ways. To date, you may have thought normal portion sizes were simply insane limits put on you. Now it's time to begin looking at exactly how much a portion size is and how you can incorporate that into your healthy, new life. For the purposes of this writing exercise, the food plan in *Why Can't I Stop Eating?* will be used. This is not to suggest that this plan is right for everyone. Rather, it is a guideline for you to use in developing a food plan that will work for you. Check with your doctor before beginning.

Breakfast: Begin by looking at the cereal boxes currently in your cabinets. On the side of the box is a suggested serving size. Write that number down, then take a measuring cup and portion out that amount. Compare the portion to what you would generally eat. What were your thoughts when you looked at the amount?

_____

_____

_____

_____

_____

_____

Lunch: Take a piece of meat or some tuna. Using a scale weigh out a three-ounce portion if you are female and a four-ounce portion if you are male. If you don't have a scale, use the palm of your hand as a general guideline. Now think about the portion you usually eat. How do the two compare? What are your thoughts about eating this amount of protein on a regular basis?

_____

_____

_____

_____

_____

_____

Dinner: Using the scale again, measure out four ounces of potato if you are female and eight if you are male. Write your thoughts regarding this portion size.

_____

_____

_____

_____

_____

_____

Am I Ready to Set Up a Food Plan?

Why not select the right role, the role of a successful
person—and rehearse it?

Maxwell Maltz

Developing a food plan is one of the first steps to making changes in your eating habits. Though you may be apprehensive or even unwilling, it is important that you consider whether you are ready to actually begin. This exercise will help you in making that determination. Remember, if you're not ready right this minute, you might be in the next. Simply write your thoughts about the questions asked.

When you think of changing your current eating habits, how do you feel? What do you fear?

_____

_____

_____

_____

_____

_____

If you want to make changes in your lifestyle, what can you do to manage these fears? Write at least ten things you are willing to do to eat healthier. For example, you will begin reading labels to see what's in the food you are eating, or you will select a leaner piece of meat at one meal. You will make a phone call rather than overeat, or you will take a short walk. Perhaps you will attend a support group meeting or begin creating a food plan.

_____   _____

_____   _____

_____   _____

_____   _____

_____   _____

Using a separate sheet of paper, write out a plan of action. For instance, where will you find a food plan? How will you go about creating guidelines for yourself? Though this may seem overwhelming, try to approach it one meal at a time. Begin with breakfast. Include a fruit, a cereal, a protein, and a dairy. Look on the cereal box and milk carton for serving sizes. For the protein, think about nonfat plain yogurt, nonfat cottage cheese, or an egg. Write out everything.

Now move on to lunch. A normal serving of protein is three ounces for a female and four ounces for a male. Generally, you will want to include two cups of vegetables and half a cup of a starchy vegetable, such as corn, peas, chickpeas, and kidney beans. At lunch you may want to include a fruit as well.

Dinner should be similar, but you may want to take out the fruit and include a fat, such as butter, margarine, or mayonnaise. Following this, you might want to include a snack. For example, a protein, a fruit, or a dairy would be a healthy snack.

Is This Really My Very Own Food Plan?

Do what most people don't do and you'll be successful.

Jim Nussbaum

You're now ready to begin developing your own food plan. Though it may seem overly strict—even obsessive—setting boundaries around the foods you eat is vital to your recovery. Many people find that without clear guidelines they simply lose momentum and find it easy to succumb to overeating. Even if you feel intimidated or unsure about creating a food plan for yourself, what have you got to lose if you simply write about it? Go ahead. Give it a try! And even though you may be afraid of failing, remember that by writing out everything and eliminating your binge foods, you are increasing your odds of succeeding. (You may want to use a separate sheet of paper to complete this exercise.)

Suggested Breakfast: 1 serving of cereal (no sugar, no flour), 1 cup of or 1 whole fruit, 1 breakfast protein (1/2 cup nonfat plain yogurt, 1/4 cup nonfat cottage cheese, 1/4 cup nonfat ricotta cheese), 1 cup skim milk. Taking this suggested breakfast plan, write out something that works for you. Once you have decided on a breakfast plan, write out one week's worth of menus. Then write your thoughts about eating these foods.

_____

_____

_____

_____

Suggested Lunch: 3 ounces protein for females (4 ounces for males), 1 cup vegetables, 1/2 cup starch (e.g., peas, corn, chickpeas), 1 cup salad or vegetables, 2 tablespoons dressing, 1 whole or 1 cup fruit. From this, construct your own lunch menu, then write out a week's worth of menus. How can you implement this plan into your life? To be successful, what will you have to change?

_____

_____

_____

_____

Suggested Dinner: 3 ounces protein for females (4 ounces for males), 1 cup vegetables, 1/2 cup starch (1 cup for males), 1 cup salad or vegetables, 2 tablespoons dressing, 1 fat (1 tablespoon whipped butter or margarine, 1 teaspoon butter or margarine, 1 teaspoon oil, or 1 teaspoon mayonnaise). Write out a week's worth of dinner menus, then write about your feelings regarding this plan.

_____

_____

_____

_____

Suggested Snack: 1 cup nonfat plain yogurt or 1 cup skim milk, 1 serving of cereal (no flour, no sugar), 1 whole or 1 cup fruit. Develop your own plan and write out seven snacks, which is a week's worth.

_____

_____

_____

What Do I Do with My Food Plan?

Freedom is a system based on courage.

Charles Péguy

In the past several exercises you have formed a clear picture of your eating habits and their effect on your life and have developed the type of food plan you need. Now it's time to think about how you will incorporate this new way of eating into your life. And though it may seem to be a contradiction, following a food plan will provide you with freedom from obsessing about food.

What do you think your biggest obstacle will be when trying to follow this plan? Why?

_____

_____

_____

_____

What can you do to overcome this and other obstacles?

_____

_____

_____

_____

It has been said that those most successful in recovering from food addiction are willing to go to any lengths to remain in recovery. A big part of recovery is following your food plan. What lengths are you prepared to go to in order to follow your plan?

_____

_____

_____

_____

_____

What lifestyle changes will you have to make to be successful? Are you willing to do this? Why or why not?

_____

_____

_____

_____

_____

What Kind of Eating Schedule Will I Have?

Don't let life discourage you; everyone who got
where he is had to begin where he was.

Richard L. Evans

Most food addicts don't have normal eating schedules but simply eat as much as they can throughout the day without any thought to developing designated meals, portion amounts, or mealtimes. Creating specific time periods to eat meals enables you to become aware of your eating habits and allows you to regulate the amount of food you eat. Even though you may feel resistant, simply pick up your pen and begin writing. With each word, you will begin to work out a much-needed schedule.

Taking into account that meals should be eaten four to five hours apart, write out specific times for breakfast, lunch, dinner, and a snack. Begin by thinking about the other commitments in your life and work around these to write down exact time periods for each meal.

_____

_____

_____

_____

_____

_____

What do you think about eating meals at specific times each day? Write your thoughts.

_____

_____

_____

_____

_____

_____

In doing this, what do you believe is your biggest obstacle? How can you over-come it?

_____

_____

_____

_____

_____

_____

What about the People I Live With?

If you judge people, you have no time to love them.

Mother Teresa

If you live with other people, changing your eating patterns may have consequences for them as well. While it is not your place to judge their eating patterns,
you must be sure that you take care of your own needs without jeopardizing your
food plan. This exercise will allow you to think about ways of incorporating your
recovery lifestyle into your home environment. If you do not live with others, you
may want to think about people in your life with whom you share meals.
Knowing what you face in various situations will help you to plan for success.

Describe your eating habits when you are with your family and/or the people with
whom you live. Be specific about past events and amounts of food eaten.

_____

_____

_____

_____

_____

_____

When you change your eating patterns, what do you believe your family will object to most?

_____

_____

_____

_____

_____

_____

Write down five specific ways that you can overcome the objections mentioned above. For instance, rather than serving dessert, suggest that your family go out for ice cream. Or rather than baking a birthday cake, you can purchase one. This will keep you away from preparing or living with foods that are dangerous to you.

_____

_____

_____

_____

_____

What about Exercise?

We must use the time as a tool not as a couch.

John F. Kennedy

Though many food addicts are overweight and have no desire to exercise, studies have shown that physical movement increases production of brain chemicals that help to alleviate stress and increase feelings of comfort. While it may be tempting to wait until you reach a certain weight, it is important to reconsider. To begin, you will need to explore your attitudes about exercise and the roadblocks you may experience. So begin writing your way to working out!

When you think about exercising, what beliefs come to your mind? How do these thoughts make you feel?

_____

_____

_____

_____

_____

_____

Describe your current physical condition and the types of exercise you are capable of doing.

_____

_____

_____

_____

_____

_____

Write about the biggest obstacle you face when exercising, then develop a way to overcome this. For example, if procrastination is most troublesome, set aside a certain time each day to exercise.

_____

_____

_____

_____

_____

_____

What about Grocery Shopping?

Self trust is the first secret of success.

Ralph Waldo Emerson

Though it may not occur to you, grocery shopping can be one of the most difficult activities you may be asked to do while in recovery. Not only are you being asked to go into a place where all of your binge foods are readily accessible, but you are also being assaulted by countless marketing techniques designed to entice you into buying more food than you may want or need. You will need to be very aware of your thoughts and feelings during the grocery shopping process. If you aren't the primary shopper in your household, there still may be times when you must go into a grocery or convenience store, so don't skip over this exercise!

Think about the last time you went into a grocery or convenience store. What feelings and thoughts did you have? Describe your experience. Be specific.

_____

_____

_____

_____

_____

_____

What is the most difficult part of grocery shopping for you? What, if anything, can you do to help overcome this?

_____

_____

_____

_____

_____

_____

Some people suggest sticking to the outside aisles of the grocery store as most fresh foods are kept there. What are your thoughts about this? Is it possible for you to do this? If so, when will you begin?

_____

_____

_____

_____

_____

_____

How Can I Eat Out?

You can have anything you want if you want it
desperately enough. You must want it with an inner
exuberance that erupts through the skin and
joins the energy that created the world.

Sheilah Graham

Similar to grocery shopping, eating out can sometimes be dangerous for food addicts. Again, you have one place where almost any type of food you may want is available. To successfully come through the eating-out experience, you will need to think about the situation a little more deeply than you may be used to. The following questions will assist you in that process.

Describe the last three times you ate out. What did you eat? How much? What were you feeling? Be specific about the amounts and types of food you ate.

_____

_____

_____

_____

_____

_____

_____

Write down three of your favorite restaurants. Using your food plan, make a list of healthy foods you can eat at each restaurant. Once again, it is necessary to be specific about the types and amounts of food.

_____

_____

_____

_____

_____

_____

Some food addicts choose to weigh and measure their food. If you decide to do this, what can you do to make it easier while eating out? If you choose not to weigh and measure your food, how will you control your portions? For example, you may choose to use a plate as a way to control your portions. A dinner plate filled with certain percentages of the food on your plan may serve to control what you eat. You may also use parts of your body to help. For instance, your palm is about the size of a healthy portion of protein. Write your plan to weigh and measure food.

_____

_____

_____

_____

_____

_____

Section Two

Emotional

How Do My Feelings Affect My Eating?

All truths are easy to understand once they are discovered;
the point is to discover them.

Galileo Galilei

Overeating may have become such a part of your life that you aren't aware of what triggers it. The physical addiction causes physical cravings, but emotional cravings can be equally as powerful. To deal with the emotional cravings, you need to discover when you are using food to nurture yourself.

For example, when you are upset, do you instantly turn to food, or is it happiness that causes you to binge? Whatever it is that triggers your overeating, it is important that you are honest as you try to discover those feelings from which you want relief. (Identifying difficult feelings is much easier if you have already gone through a twenty-one-day withdrawal period from sugar and flour, but if not, it is still possible to do.)

To begin, in the first column on the following page, write how you felt before each of the meals listed. In the second column write about how your feelings affected each meal. Think about whether you over- or underate, if you ate very quickly, what types of food choices you made, your state of mind about the food you ate, and/or your actions toward other people.

Photocopy the following page and complete the form over three or four days. Do you notice that you consistently feel a certain way at the same time each day? Even more, do you overeat or think intensely about food to help you get through these feelings? If so, write about these patterns.

For now, don't worry about how to change the patterns. The next exercise will help you with this. The most important thing for you to do right now is to notice the patterns. Remember that this may take some time and effort on your part as most food addicts aren't used to examining their eating patterns in such a manner. Just begin writing about your feelings before each meal, then go back and read over your notes to look for patterns. No matter how tempting it is to try and analyze your writing as you go along, resist the temptation. It will be much easier to identify patterns in your behavior if you freely express your feelings by writing.

	How I felt:	How it affected my meal:
Before breakfast:	_____	_____
	_____	_____
Before lunch:	_____	_____
	_____	_____
Before dinner:	_____	_____
	_____	_____
Before snack:	_____	_____
	_____	_____

What patterns do I notice?

_____

_____

How do my emotions affect my eating patterns?

_____

_____

How Do I Nurture Myself without Overeating?

Happiness is a choice that requires effort at times.

Anonymous

In the previous exercise, you wrote about how your feelings affected your overeating. Taking these discoveries into consideration, you will now need to develop new ways of dealing with your feelings.

If you have difficulty answering the following questions, you may want to take a day or two to think them over. However, be sure to come back and write your answers.

Make a list of things you enjoy doing that do not involve buying, eating, or cooking food. Write as many as you can.

_____

_____

_____

_____

_____

_____

_____

_____

Now divide this list into two columns as shown below. After adding all the items from your list, check to see if you have at least three or four in each column. If not, add to the columns.

Quick Activities   More Involved Activities

_____   _____

_____   _____

_____   _____

_____   _____

Review the information from the previous exercise regarding your feelings before meals. Write about how you can use these quick or more involved activities during the times when you most want to eat.

_____

_____

_____

_____

Now develop a plan to help you when you feel like eating. What is the first thing you will do? The second? If you are most comfortable with taking a walk when you feel like eating, then you should write that first. If walking isn't possible, your second plan of action may involve making a phone call or writing in your journal. Whatever it is, write it down.

_____

_____

_____

_____

What's My Motivation?

Every failure is a step to success.

William Whewell

Most food addicts have experienced many failed weight-loss attempts. Because of this, beginning a new program can be traumatic or filled with dread. You need a strong, compelling reason to begin a new program. While this exercise will help you to do this, it's important that you reread what you have written on a regular basis so that your motivations are clearly in your mind when you feel weak or tempted. As always, your honesty is the most important tool you have in your recovery box.

Write down three negative experiences you have had because of your body size or your eating behavior. Next to each, write about how you felt.

_____

_____

_____

_____

_____

_____

_____

_____

Do the experiences you mentioned motivate you enough to want to follow a food plan? Explain.

_____

_____

_____

_____

_____

_____

Write down ten benefits you will gain from eating healthy and following a food plan. How important are these things to you?

_____	_____
_____	_____
_____	_____
_____	_____
_____	_____

_____

_____

_____

_____

_____

How Can I Feel Better?

Discipline is the basic set of tools we require to solve life's
problems. Without discipline we can solve nothing. With
only some discipline we can solve only some problems.
With total discipline we can solve all problems.

M. Scott Peck

If you're unaccustomed to dealing with emotions, eating becomes a way of sooth-
ing unpleasant and even pleasant feelings. Being in recovery means developing
new behavioral patterns and learning ways of coping that don't involve overeating. Though it may seem difficult at first, the more you behave in a healthy way,
the easier it will become. The key is to exercise loving discipline with yourself.
While some of us have grown to see discipline as something negative, it can be
just the opposite. Discipline with love can help you to establish lifelong healthy
eating habits. So try to keep an open mind as you write.

Write about the last experience in which you used food to soothe yourself. List the
amounts and types of food you ate and then describe your feelings.

_____

_____

_____

_____

_____

Write about an experience that did not involve food or eating when you felt soothed after being emotionally upset.

_____

_____

_____

_____

_____

_____

_____

_____

List several ways that you can soothe yourself without using food. Are you willing to use at least one of these methods? Why or why not?

_____

_____

_____

_____

_____

_____

_____

_____

_____

Am I Ready to Say Good-bye?

When one door of happiness closes, another opens;
but often we look so long at the closed door that we
do not see the one which has opened for us.

Helen Keller

Saying good-bye to food is perhaps one of the most difficult tasks a recovering food addict needs to face. While it is not possible to stop eating completely, it will be absolutely necessary to say good-bye to your binge foods if you want to recover. At first, it may seem silly, but think about the important role food has played in your life. Saying good-bye to food may cause more sadness than you expect as you will be grieving the loss of your substance. All change brings grief to some extent, but once you have gone through the process, you will discover that another door of happiness will open. So begin writing and see what you discover.

Make a list of the foods you most need to say good-bye to in order to move on in your recovery.

_____

_____

_____

_____

_____

_____

Write about your feelings when you think of saying good-bye to these foods.

_____

_____

_____

_____

_____

_____

Write a good-bye letter to these foods. Use another sheet of paper if necessary.

_____

_____

_____

_____

_____

_____

Now make a list of all the things you will gain by saying good-bye to your binge foods.

_____

_____

_____

_____

_____

_____

How Serious Is My Problem?

Our doubts are traitors and make us lose the good we oft
might win by fearing to attempt.

William Shakespeare

Being concerned about your eating behavior and knowing the extent of your problem are two very different things. If you approach your overeating as a little problem that will go away, you run the danger of not putting enough effort into your recovery, which will eventually lead you right back to where you started. This exercise will help you to determine exactly what your beliefs are.

Exactly how serious do you think your overeating problem is? Explain.

_____

_____

_____

_____

_____

_____

_____

_____

Make a list of overeating experiences that lead you to believe your problem might be more serious than you first thought.

_____

_____

_____

_____

_____

_____

_____

_____

Substitute the word *drinking* for *overeating* in the previous questions and answers that you wrote. If your eating behavior involved alcohol rather than food, would you consider the problem to be serious? Why or why not?

_____

_____

_____

_____

_____

_____

_____

_____

How Do I Feel about Setting Food Boundaries?

Even if you're on the right track, you'll get
run over if you just sit there.

Will Rogers

Food plays a very important part in our society. We use food to celebrate birth-days, anniversaries, holidays, even graduations. Unfortunately, most of the food at our celebrations is unhealthy. Because of the wide availability of food, it may become necessary for you to set boundaries about the types and amounts of food you will eat.

Though setting boundaries in public may seem overwhelming, remember that many times it's possible to get lost in the crowd. No one is monitoring your food intake. If you are asked, you can simply say no thanks. You may want to add that the type of food you were offered doesn't agree with you. Another option is to say that you have medical reasons for not eating that type of food. In general, most people are not rude enough to pry into your personal life. If you are asked further, you can simply say that you prefer not to discuss it.

Are there people in your life who would feel disappointed if you refused to eat the food they offered you? If so, make a list of these people.

_____

_____

_____

_____

_____

How would you feel about refusing to eat the food they prepared? Explain.

_____

_____

_____

_____

_____

To make saying no easier, some overeaters use truthful excuses. For example, a person physically addicted to sugar and flour might say that he or she has medical reasons for not eating certain foods. Can you think of four such excuses that would work in your life? Write them down.

_____

_____

_____

_____

_____

_____

Write about how it would feel to use these excuses. What could you do to make it easier?

_____

_____

_____

_____

_____

Is Food Love?

We must do the best we can with what we have.

Edward Rowland Sill

The only way some food addicts know how to express love is either to eat food prepared by others or to prepare food for others. This may not be a conscious decision, but think about how often you have felt either rejected when someone else wouldn't eat what you so lovingly prepared or guilty for turning down food that was made especially for you. This exercise will help you discover to what extent you use food to show and feel love, as well as provide you with some ideas to change these behavior patterns.

As a child and later into adulthood, what do you remember about food being used to show love in your family? Write about three specific incidents.

_____

_____

_____

_____

_____

_____

_____

_____

_____

What types of foods do you associate with love and feeling loved? Name the individuals with whom you link these foods. Be specific.

_____

_____

_____

_____

_____

_____

_____

_____

_____

Make a list of ten ways that you can show love without using food or eating. When you have done this, list ten ways you can feel loved without using food or eating.

_____	_____
_____	_____
_____	_____
_____	_____
_____	_____
_____	_____
_____	_____
_____	_____
_____	_____

Do I Use Food to Celebrate?

Welcome anything that comes to you,
but do not long for anything else.

André Gide

In the same way that food can be used to show love, it is also used as a means of celebration. So many of our special events have special foods available. The danger for food addicts is that they are consumed by the food to the point of not caring about the special event. Knowing exactly how you use food is an important step toward recovery.

Think about the last four celebrations you attended. How important to you were the types and/or amounts of food available at these events? If you were responsible for preparing any of the food, how much time and effort did you put in?

_____

_____

_____

_____

_____

_____

_____

_____

Have you ever had a celebration that didn't involve food? If so, write about it. Then write about your feelings when you think of attending a celebration where food is not available.

_____

_____

_____

_____

_____

Make a list of ten ways you can celebrate without using food. Then choose one and write about the next time you can use it.

_____ _____

_____ _____

_____ _____

_____ _____

_____ _____

_____

_____

_____

_____

Is Food Fun?

Humor is emotional chaos remembered in
times of tranquility.

James Thurber

Food addicts also use food as a means of having fun. Because many people have overeaten from childhood, learning to enjoy life without food is challenging. Writing about fun may be one of the most difficult things you are asked to do in your recovery. Though you may be tempted to skip over this exercise for a more "serious" topic, keep in mind that having fun is just as important to your recovery as anything else.

Write about a time in your life when you had fun without food being involved. Be specific about what you were doing and how it felt. If you can't recall having any good times without food, write about what it feels like to not have fun without food.

_____

_____

_____

_____

_____

_____

_____

As a child, what hobbies or interests did you have? Write about the joy you experienced from these. What did it feel like to be so involved in an activity?

_____

_____

_____

_____

_____

_____

_____

Make a list of ten ways in which you could have fun without food. Make them realistic for you and your life. Then put a star next to the one you are willing to try over the next few days.

_____

_____

_____

_____

_____

_____

_____

_____

_____

_____

_____

Is Food Comfort?

Believe that you are bigger than your difficulties,
for you are, indeed.

Norman Vincent Peale

While you may be aware that food is a means of comforting yourself, you may not realize exactly how often or to what degree you use food. This exercise is designed to provide you with further awareness.

Write about three incidents when you used food to comfort yourself. (If you're an adult, write about one from your childhood, one from your teenage years, and one from adulthood.) Give as many details as you possibly can about the events, your feelings, and the types and amounts of foods you ate.

_____

_____

_____

_____

_____

_____

_____

_____

Now take each of these incidents and write about another way you could have comforted yourself. Once again, be specific.

_____

_____

_____

_____

_____

_____

_____

_____

_____

Combining everything that you have discovered in the last two questions, write out a plan for how to comfort yourself from now on. Be sure that this plan does not involve food or eating. Write a sentence in which you commit to use this plan.

_____

_____

_____

_____

_____

_____

_____

_____

_____

Do I Have Eating Buddies?

The only abnormality is the incapacity to love.

Anaïs Nin

Though your first reaction to the question above may be to deny that you have eating buddies, it is a good idea to think deeply about this issue. Since, in general, people who share common interests are attracted to each other, it is not unreasonable to assume that one or two of your friends or family members may be as preoccupied with food as you are. It's also necessary to realize that simply because some people in your life may be your eating buddies, you don't necessarily need to isolate from them. Being aware of the roles people play in your life allows you to plan to take care of yourself more effectively. It does not force you to push these people out of your life.

Is there someone in your life with whom you overeat? Is there someone with whom you regularly talk about food or losing weight? Write about three specific incidents when you have overeaten or discussed weight loss with this person.

_____

_____

_____

_____

_____

_____

Write about four people in your life and the interests/activities you have in common.

_____

_____

_____

_____

_____

_____

_____

_____

_____

Is there someone in your life with whom you do not overeat and/or discuss weight? If so, write about this person. If not, write about where you may find someone like this.

_____

_____

_____

_____

_____

_____

_____

_____

Do I Have Hope?

Man is what he believes.

Anton Chekhov

Being hopeful is perhaps one of the most difficult things for a food addict. Accustomed to seeing the negative side of things and failing many weight-loss attempts, food addicts are often unable to feel hopeful without great effort. Yet believing that it is possible for life to get better is an important part of recovery. So even though you may not believe that you can recover, why not at least be open to the possibility?

Do you have hope that you can get and stay in recovery? That you will be a healthy weight? That your eating habits will improve? Explain.

_____

_____

_____

_____

_____

_____

_____

Write about the last few times that you had hope of recovering from your addiction. What happened?

_____

_____

_____

_____

_____

_____

_____

Are you willing to believe that recovery is possible for you? Why or why not? Be specific.

_____

_____

_____

_____

_____

_____

Is Eating Tied into My Identity?

Only the shallow know themselves.

Oscar Wilde

For many food addicts eating is not only a large part of daily life but is deeply connected to how they view themselves—to their identity. For many food addicts, eating is all they've ever known. Letting go of this idea can sometimes be challenging.

Use the space below to write about how you see yourself. What is your identity? Who are you? What do you like to do? What are your beliefs? Your accomplishments? Your passions? Be specific.

_____

_____

_____

_____

_____

_____

_____

_____

_____

_____

_____

Now use the space below to write about who you would like to be. How do you want others to perceive you? Do you want to be shy or outgoing, physically active, social, funny, and so on? Once again, be specific.

_____

_____

_____

_____

_____

_____

_____

_____

_____

_____

_____

Am I Safe?

The handwriting on the wall may be a forgery.

Ralph Hodgson

By now you are very aware of the many ways in which you have used food, but one that is often overlooked involves safety. For many food addicts, being overweight serves as protection, almost a sort of body armor, against the world. In order to recover, you will need to be aware of both your fears and the role your body size plays in alleviating them. Even if you don't think this is a problem for you, write anyway.

How often do you feel unsafe? Write about three events. Be sure to include the specific foods you ate during this time.

_____

_____

_____

_____

_____

_____

_____

_____

_____

How do you feel about the idea that your body size may be a means of protection from the world? Explain.

_____

_____

_____

_____

_____

_____

_____

Make a list of five ways you feel safe that don't involve food.

_____

_____

_____

_____

_____

_____

_____

_____

_____

_____

_____

Who Will Support Me?

I can't give you a sure-fire formula for success,
but I can give you a formula for failure: try to
please everybody all the time.

Herbert Bayard Swope

One of the biggest contributors to success in recovery is the development of a network of people who will support you in your recovery. In the previous section, you wrote about one person who you could turn to for help if you needed it. Though this is a good beginning, you will need to develop more friends, as it is unfair to depend on one person for everything.

Make a list of all the people in your life who you believe would support the changes you are planning to or have already made. Next to each write why you believe he or she is someone who would help you.

_____

_____

_____

_____

_____

_____

_____

Now write down ten places where you could meet people who would be supportive of your healthy lifestyle. Include places you do not currently go.

_____

_____

_____

_____

_____

_____

_____

_____

_____

_____

How do you feel about reaching out to other people you don't know? Explain. Are you willing to try? Why or why not?

_____

_____

_____

_____

_____

_____

_____

_____

What If I Fail?

Notice the difference between what happens when a
man says to himself, "I have failed three times" and what
happens when he says, "I am a failure."

S. I. Hayakawa

Fear of failing prevents many people from taking action. Accustomed to unsuccessful dieting attempts, most food addicts are disillusioned, even bitter, about once again attempting something that has seemed to be impossible. This exercise will help you to determine your beliefs about success and failure.

What does it mean to you to be successful? Explain where these beliefs come from.

_____

_____

_____

_____

_____

_____

_____

_____

_____

_____

What does it mean to you to be a failure? Where do these beliefs come from? Explain.

_____

_____

_____

_____

_____

_____

_____

Explain how these beliefs fit or don't fit into your life and recovery today. Do you accept them as being true? Why or not?

_____

_____

_____

_____

_____

_____

_____

How Do I Feel about My New Behaviors?

Success is the failure of many a man.

Cindy Adams

If you've been using this journal in order, then by now you may have experienced some success. Even if it isn't perfect or exactly the way you may want it, you are most likely making progress in your recovery. Remember that progress does not have to involve weight loss. It can be something spiritual or emotional, such as accepting that you have a problem. With many of these writing exercises completed, it is time to look at your experience thus far.

Make a list of what you are doing differently since first beginning this journal. Remember to include attitude and behavioral changes as well as eating and exercise adjustments. Next to each change write a word to describe how you feel about the change.

_____

_____

_____

_____

_____

_____

_____

Now take four of the changes you mentioned and write about each experience. Give as many details as possible about your feelings and thoughts while doing these things.

_____

_____

_____

_____

_____

_____

_____

_____

_____

_____

_____

_____

How many of your behavioral changes do you consider to be successful? Why do you consider each a success? If you feel you haven't been successful, what could you do to change the results?

_____

_____

_____

_____

_____

What Are My Eating Rituals?

The game of life is not so much holding a
good hand as playing a poor one well.

H. T. Leslie

A big part of overeating for most food addicts involves what are known as eating rituals. These are habits or activities that are performed regularly while overeating. For some, a ritual is as simple as watching television while eating. For others, a ritual can be something as exacting as eating yellow M&M's while reading *Time* magazine. Each person's rituals are different and unique to his or her environment.

When you think about eating your favorite foods, what activity or nonactivity goes along with this? Be specific about which food goes with what experience.

_____

_____

_____

_____

_____

_____

When was the last time you did the activities you described without eating? If you've never done this, write about what it would be like to not eat during these activities. If you have done this, write about the experience.

_____

_____

_____

_____

_____

_____

How do these eating rituals affect your eating behavior? Do you feel as if you can live without eating those foods? Can you live without doing these activities? Explain.

_____

_____

_____

_____

_____

_____

Why Is It So Difficult?

I do not know anyone who has gotten to the top without
hard work. That is the recipe. It will not always get you
to the top, but it should get you pretty near.

Margaret Thatcher

While working your recovery program, there may be times when you feel overwhelmed and tired. Though this is normal, it can be a threat to the healthy lifestyle you have begun developing. This exercise will help you to be aware of your feelings and to develop a plan to manage them.

What is the most difficult part of working a recovery program? Why is it so difficult? How do you feel about needing to work the program even though it is challenging?

_____

_____

_____

_____

_____

_____

When you have a difficult project to complete at work or at home, what steps do you take to make it manageable so that you can successfully finish? Explain.

_____

_____

_____

_____

_____

_____

_____

Take the steps you described and write about how you can use them to make aspects of your recovery easier. Be sure that your ideas do not decrease the quality of your recovery.

_____

_____

_____

_____

_____

_____

_____

Section Three

Spiritual

What Do I Believe?

I would never die for my beliefs because I might be wrong.

Bertrand Russell

In general, food addicts can sometimes have negative attitudes about life and their abilities. After years of trying to stop overeating and failing, many have come to doubt the general goodness of the world. To help develop new and healthier beliefs, it is first necessary to examine what you currently believe. As always, be as honest as you possibly can. Try not to judge your beliefs. Simply remind yourself that the first step to changing something is acknowledging your current situation.

Write ten words that come to mind when you hear the word *spirituality*.

_____ _____

_____ _____

_____ _____

_____ _____

_____ _____

Do you consider yourself a spiritual person? Why or why not?

_____

_____

_____

_____

_____

_____

As a child, what were you taught about religion? About spirituality?

_____

_____

_____

_____

_____

_____

Do you still believe these things today? Write about what you believe.

_____

_____

_____

_____

_____

_____

What's a Higher Power?

If you can't have faith in what is held up to you for faith,
you must find things to believe in yourself, for a life without
faith in something is too narrow a space to live.

George E. Woodberry

Having faith in something outside of yourself is for some people a challenging aspect of recovery. This belief can be in God, Allah, the energy, or even the support at a group meeting. After many failed dieting attempts, most food addicts have difficulty believing that a power greater than themselves exists, much less cares about them. Though it may not seem important to you, or may require a huge leap of faith, a belief in a power greater than yourself provides you with assistance when you are experiencing difficult times in your recovery and life in general. Countless addicts in recovery will attest to this. This exercise will help you to discover your Higher Power as you understand it.

When you think of a Higher Power, what comes into your mind? Explain. What are your beliefs about having a Higher Power?

_____

_____

_____

_____

_____

Are you willing to believe in a power greater than yourself? Why or why not? If you don't believe in anything, is there a small step you can take to discover something that will work for you? Explain.

_____

_____

_____

_____

_____

_____

_____

If you had a Higher Power, what would he, she, or it be like? Be specific about the role this Higher Power would play in your life and the characteristics he, she, or it would have.

_____

_____

_____

_____

_____

_____

_____

What Is Spirituality?

To believe in God or in a guiding force because someone
tells you to is the height of stupidity. We are given senses to
receive our information within. With our own eyes we see,
and with our own skin we feel. With our intelligence,
it is intended that we understand. But each person
must puzzle it out for himself or herself.

Sophy Burnham

Many food addicts confuse spirituality with religion. Though they may appear to
be the same, the difference is that spirituality does not demand that certain rituals and/or beliefs be practiced, nor does it require attendance or even organized
mandates. Spirituality is a very personal belief in the general goodness of someone or something that guides the universe, while religion is the observance of certain practices devoted to the reflection of unified beliefs. In this exercise, you will
explore your spiritual beliefs.

Write a definition of the word *spirituality* as it manifests itself in your life.

_____

_____

_____

_____

_____

Take a few moments and look outside. Or if you have time, go to the beach, the park, the mountains, or a flower garden. Write about what you see and then relate this to the idea that a higher being is responsible for everything you are looking at.

_____

_____

_____

_____

_____

_____

Reread your definition of spirituality. Do you feel you are spiritual? Explain. If not, what is standing in your way and how can you get through it?

_____

_____

_____

_____

_____

_____

Am I Religious?

Say nothing of my religion. It is known to God and myself
alone. Its evidence before the world is to be sought in
my life: if it has been honest and dutiful to society the
religion which has regulated it cannot be a bad one.

Thomas Jefferson

While spirituality is an important part of recovery, whether you choose to partici-
pate in religious activities is up to you. This exercise will help you to determine
where your current religious practices, if any, fit into your food addiction recovery. Many food addicts have simply accepted the religious practices they were
raised with, but as with everything in your new life, it's worth taking a look at
whether they work for you today.

Write a definition of the word *religion* as it manifests itself in your life.

_____

_____

_____

_____

_____

_____

Make a list of five things you believe about religion.

_____

_____

_____

_____

_____

_____

_____

_____

_____

Explain how these beliefs fit or don't fit into your recovery plan. If they don't fit, what can you do? Explain.

_____

_____

_____

_____

_____

_____

Who's in Charge?

Pray as if everything depended upon God and work
as if everything depended upon man.

Cardinal Francis Spellman

Sometimes the only way that we actually achieve serenity in our lives is to give up control of those things we cannot change. For many, this goes against the way we were raised. Yet trying to control the uncontrollable only causes us pain and frustration. The following exercises will assist you in recognizing the things over which you are powerless.

What means have you used to control the outcome of events in your life? Name at least five and be specific. For example, have you lied about something to get your way or have you bullied someone into doing something that he or she didn't want to?

_____

_____

_____

_____

_____

_____

_____

_____

Looking back on the events you wrote about in the previous question, did the methods you used to control things work? Why or why not? Would you be willing to change your behavior? If so, how? If not, why?

_____

_____

_____

_____

_____

_____

_____

Now looking at your answer to the question above, write about the idea that you could ask a Higher Power to help you with your recovery.

_____

_____

_____

_____

_____

_____

_____

Am I Angry at God?

I have too much respect for the idea of God to make
it responsible for such an absurd world.

Georges Duhamel

After many failed dieting attempts, many food addicts become angry with God.
While the thought of being angry at your Higher Power may be frightening to
you, denying the feeling can be even more dangerous. Stored up feelings of anger
and resentment can become excuses to overeat. Dealing with these feelings will be
necessary for you to proceed in your recovery.

When you think of the concept of God, how do you feel? Explain.

_____

_____

_____

_____

_____

_____

_____

Name four events in your life when you felt angry with God. Be specific.

_____

_____

_____

_____

_____

_____

_____

_____

_____

_____

_____

What do you think will happen if you are angry with God? Is this realistic? Explain.

_____

_____

_____

_____

_____

_____

_____

_____

_____

_____

Do I Believe Things Will Be Okay?

A spiritually optimistic point of view holds that the
universe is woven out of a fabric of love. Everything that is
happening is ultimately for the good if we're willing to face
it head-on and use our adversities for soul growth.

Joan Borysenko

Part of living a spiritual life means believing in the general goodness of the world.
Though sometimes believing that all is as it should be can be a challenge, it can
provide a great deal of comfort. Even if this concept is completely unfamiliar to
you, work through this exercise and explore your beliefs.

When you look back on your life, can you think of some things that worked out
differently than you had hoped but that you now know were for the best? Explain.

_____

_____

_____

_____

_____

_____

Are there things in your life that you believe worked out better than you could
have ever planned? Explain.

_____

_____

_____

_____

_____

_____

Do you believe that things will work out even if you can't see it at the time?
Explain. How does this relate to your recovery?

_____

_____

_____

_____

_____

_____

_____

What Did I Believe in the Past?

Every man is the creature of the age in which he lives; very
few are able to raise themselves above the ideas of the time.

Voltaire

As a child, along with many other things, you inherited the religious beliefs of your
family of origin. Maybe you've never taken the time to think deeply about these beliefs, but it is possible that they are strongly affecting your life today whether you
are aware of it or not. Take some time to examine your past beliefs about religion,
as they are most likely tied to your feelings about spirituality today.

List what you think of when you hear the word *religion,* then make another list
about *spirituality.* Write about your earliest memories involving religion, church,
and spirituality. Describe as many as you possibly can. If you did not have a religious upbringing, write what your feelings are about religion.

Reread the answer you wrote for the previous question. How do these memories affect you today? Explain.

_____

_____

_____

_____

_____

_____

If you could change one aspect of your spiritual life today, what would it be? Is this change related to your childhood beliefs? Explain.

_____

_____

_____

_____

_____

_____

_____

What Do I Believe Now?

The imagination imitates.
It is the critical spirit that creates.

Oscar Wilde

Though you have already done some writing about your beliefs, it's important to continue as deepening your spirituality requires that you regularly examine your beliefs. Most times writing further on a subject increases your understanding and knowledge in that area. If you repeat something you've already written, there's no harm in that. So keep writing!

Make a list of ten things you believe about your spirituality at this moment.

_____

_____

_____

_____

_____

_____

_____

_____

_____

_____

Now take the three strongest beliefs you have and determine whether they are helpful to your recovery. Explain your reasons for each one.

_____

_____

_____

_____

_____

_____

_____

_____

_____

How do your spiritual beliefs affect your food addiction recovery today? Give details and be specific.

_____

_____

_____

_____

_____

_____

_____

_____

What Do I Want to Believe?

We do not do well except when we know where the best is
and when we have touched it and hold its power within us.

Joseph Joubert

Now that you have considered how your spiritual beliefs are important to your recovery, you may want to write about what you'd like to believe. Sometimes simply by writing down your hopes and dreams, you take the first step to making them a reality.

Find a prayer, poem, inspirational quote, or song that has special meaning to you. What about it do you like? Can you relate the ideas to your spirituality? Explain.

_____

_____

_____

_____

_____

_____

_____

_____

_____

Take the ideas from your reading and expand them so they are personal to you.
How can you use these ideas to help your recovery?

_____

_____

_____

_____

_____

_____

Make a list of ten things you'd like to believe in the future. How likely do you think
it is that you will come to believe them? Explain.

_____

_____

_____

_____

_____

_____

_____

_____

_____

_____

Am I Ready to Do the Footwork?

Whatever God's dream about man may be, it seems certain
it cannot come true unless man cooperates.

Stella Terrill Mann

Throughout the years, many food addicts have asked God for help in losing weight, yet they continued to overeat. While your Higher Power is willing to help you in your recovery efforts, it is necessary for you to do your part, known as the footwork, in order to be successful. This exercise will help you to recognize some of the footwork you need to do.

Do you believe it is your Higher Power's will for you to be abstinent and work your recovery program? Explain.

_____

_____

_____

_____

_____

_____

Make a list of the things you need to do to be in recovery. Next to each write how your Higher Power can help you. Be specific.

_____

_____

_____

_____

_____

_____

_____

Many food addicts say a special prayer or ask for help when they feel like overeating. Write your prayer here. Can you make a commitment to use these words when you feel like overeating? Explain.

_____

_____

_____

_____

_____

_____

_____

Am I Humble?

If I only had a little humility, I'd be perfect.

Ted Turner

Humility is known as the state of being humble, which is the lack of arrogance and pride. Those who are prideful or arrogant have no room in their lives for a Higher Power who knows more than they do. Prideful or arrogant people believe that they are the ultimate authority about nearly everything. Humble people, on the other hand, are open and willing to hear suggestions from others and make changes if necessary. Take some time to examine your humility.

Define humility. How humble do you think you are? Give five specific examples to prove your point.

_____

_____

_____

_____

_____

_____

_____

_____

_____

Recognizing that a humble person is open to suggestions, write about what this means in your life. Are you willing to listen to other people, or do you believe you know everything you need to know to recover?

_____

_____

_____

_____

_____

_____

_____

It has been said that if you think you are humble, then you are not. How do you feel about this? How do your feelings relate to what you've written in this exercise? Explain.

_____

_____

_____

_____

_____

_____

_____

Am I Grateful?

Gratitude is born in hearts that take time
to count up past mercies.

Charles E. Jefferson

A big part of recovery is acknowledging what you have in your life. As is the case with most addicts, concentrating on what appear to be the negative aspects has become a habit. Helping yourself to become aware of how many good things you actually have in your life will deepen your spirituality and enhance your connection with your Higher Power.

Make a list of twenty things you are grateful for. Be sure to find twenty.

_____   _____

_____   _____

_____   _____

_____   _____

_____   _____

_____   _____

_____   _____

_____   _____

_____   _____

_____   _____

Now list five negative aspects in your life that you could begin to think of as good aspects.

_____

_____

_____

_____

_____

_____

Reread the previous list. How do you feel about what you've written? Explain.

_____

_____

_____

_____

_____

_____

How would your life be different if every day you thanked your Higher Power for one thing? Are you willing to do this? Explain.

_____

_____

_____

_____

_____

_____

Do I Have a Special Object?

Getting ahead in a difficult profession requires avid
faith in yourself. That is why some people with mediocre
talent, but with great inner drive, go much further
than people with vastly superior talent.

Sophia Loren

Some food addicts find that having a special object helps them to connect to their Higher Power and to believe in themselves. Though it may take a little work to think of something that's special to you, it will be worth the effort, especially during very difficult times. Begin writing and discover your special object. Don't try to find the perfect object. Instead think of things around you such as a piece of jewelry, a statue, a book, and so on.

Name ten objects that are important to you. Next to each write why it is important and what it represents.

_____   _____

_____   _____

_____   _____

_____   _____

_____   _____

If you had to choose one of these things to be your special object, which one would it be? Why?

_____

_____

_____

_____

_____

Does the object you chose fit with the spirit of your recovery? Explain. If not, choose an object that does. Are you willing to hold this object when you feel like overeating? Why or why not?

_____

_____

_____

_____

_____

What's a God Box?

They say that God is everywhere, and yet we always
think of Him as somewhat of a recluse.

Emily Dickinson

Similar to your special object, a God box will also assist you in deepening your relationship with your Higher Power and learning to ask for help. Think of this as the physical representation of your prayers for help. To begin, find a box of your choice. It can be any size or shape, just so it feels right to you.

Make a list of twenty things that you would like your Higher Power to help you with.

_____   _____

_____   _____

_____   _____

_____   _____

_____   _____

_____   _____

_____   _____

_____   _____

_____   _____

_____   _____

Rewrite each of these twenty things on its own piece of paper. Now say each one out loud, fold it up, and put it in the box. When you are done, ask your Higher Power to help you with these things. Write about how it felt to do this.

_____

_____

_____

_____

_____

_____

_____

_____

Are you willing to use your God box in the future? Explain. Do you think your God box will help you in your recovery? Why or why not?

_____

_____

_____

_____

_____

_____

_____

_____

_____

_____

Can I Accept My Life the Way It Is?

This art of resting the mind and the power of dismissing
from it all care and worry is probably one of the
secrets of energy in our great men.

Captain J. A. Hadfield

Part of believing in a Higher Power and living a spiritual life is accepting that certain circumstances in your life are out of your control no matter how much you struggle. For example, the fact that you are a food addict is something you had no say in, but whether you work your recovery program is something you do have control over. This exercise will help you in accepting those things that are beyond your control. When you are able to achieve this on a regular basis, you will be able to rest your mind and lessen your cares and worries.

Write down ten things in your personal life that are beyond your control.

_____   _____

_____   _____

_____   _____

_____   _____

_____   _____

Now take each item from the previous list and write how you feel about being
unable to control the outcome of each.

_____

_____

_____

_____

_____

_____

_____

_____

_____

_____

What would happen if you made a decision to accept these things as part of your
life for today? Explain. Do these ideas fit in with your recovery program? Why or
why not?

_____

_____

_____

Do I Have the Courage to Change?

Courage is resistance to fear, mastery of fear—
not absence of fear.

Mark Twain

Just the thought of making changes can sometimes send chills up your spine. Yet without changes, sometimes even drastic ones, you will not be able to progress in your recovery. And though you may be afraid, you can move ahead anyway. This exercise will help you to determine your thoughts and feelings about change.

When you think of making changes in your lifestyle to support your recovery, how do you feel? Explain.

_____

_____

_____

_____

_____

_____

_____

Make a list of ten changes you would like to make in your life right now.

_____

_____

_____

_____

_____

_____

_____

_____

_____

_____

Reread your list and then determine the two most important changes you'd like to make. Are these desires realistic? If so, how can you go about making these changes? If not, choose two that are realistic and write a plan to begin the process.

_____

_____

_____

_____

_____

_____

_____

Do I Have the Wisdom to Know the Difference?

We don't receive wisdom; we must discover it for ourselves
after a journey that no one can take us on or spare us.

Marcel Proust

Often it is not easy to know the difference between the things you can change and those you cannot. This is where wisdom comes in. Wisdom helps you to determine the difference between the two. Yet how you get wise is often a mystery to most people. Writing out this exercise will assist you on your journey toward the answers you seek.

In the previous two exercises you wrote about things you need to accept and things you need to change. Go back over your lists and fill in the two columns below.

Things I Can Change   Things I Cannot Change

_____   _____

_____   _____

_____   _____

_____   _____

_____   _____

_____   _____

_____   _____

Now look at each column once again. In the "Things I Can Change" column, write down at least one way you can begin making the changes you listed. Use the space below to write about how you feel when you think of making these changes.

_____

_____

_____

_____

_____

_____

_____

Now take what you have written in the "Things I Cannot Change" column and write how you can begin to accept that, for today, these are part of your life. How does it feel to be unable to change these things? Explain.

_____

_____

_____

_____

_____

_____

_____

Does My Higher Power Care about My Recovery?

I know God will not give me anything I can't handle.
I just wish He didn't trust me so much.

Mother Teresa

Many food addicts find it unbelievable that their Higher Power actually cares about something so seemingly small in the universe as their food addiction recovery. Though it is tempting to think this, it is important to realize that this attitude could also serve as an excuse for inaction. After all, if God doesn't care about your recovery, then why should you? Before coming to any conclusions, take some time to examine your beliefs.

Pretend that God does care about your recovery. Write about what you would do differently. Why? If you already believe that God cares about your recovery, then write about how you can deepen your relationship in this area.

_____

_____

_____

_____

_____

_____

_____

_____

Now write a letter to God asking for help with your recovery. Be specific about what you need and what you'd like, but remember not to give instructions. Rather, ask for help. (Use a separate sheet of paper if necessary.)

_____

_____

_____

_____

_____

_____

_____

_____

How did it feel to write the letter and ask for help? Explain. Do you believe this help will come to you? Why or why not?

_____

_____

_____

_____

_____

_____

_____

_____

_____

Do I Believe That Everything Will Be Okay?

Don't fall victim to your own melodrama. Keep things
in perspective. The odds are that your problem is solvable.
Address the solution and don't dwell on the problem
to the point at which it paralyzes you.

Harvey Mackay

A deep belief in the positive power of the universe will go a long way in helping you to deal with life without overeating. In other words, if you know that things will work out, then you won't need to overeat to make them better. But as much as you may like to, you can't force yourself to believe. You can, however, make an effort to stop doubting.

Think back over your life. Try to remember three times when you wanted something very badly but didn't get it. What happened? How do you feel today about not getting these things? Explain.

_____

_____

_____

_____

_____

_____

_____

Imagine your life today if you had gotten these things. Where would you be? Who would you be with? What would the quality of your life be?

_____

_____

_____

_____

_____

_____

How can you use these experiences to help you with a problem you may have today or in the future? Explain.

_____

_____

_____

_____

_____

_____

What Have I Learned?

An unexamined life is not worth living.

Socrates

Now that you've come to the end of this book, it's time to examine what you've learned during this process. Before you begin writing, go back and read several entries from each section.

Make a list of five things you've learned about the physical aspects of food addiction.

_____

_____

_____

_____

_____

Make a list of five things you've learned about the emotional aspects of food addiction.

_____

_____

_____

_____

_____

Make a list of five things you've learned about the spiritual aspects of food addiction.

_____

_____

_____

_____

_____

Write about how you can use these things to improve your life. Then make a list of five things you plan to accomplish over the next several weeks as you continue your recovery.

_____

_____

_____

_____

_____

Notes

1. M. White and D. Epston, *Narrative Means to Therapeutic Ends* (New York: Norton, 1990), 36.

2. T. Vance, *Letters Home* (New York: Pantheon Books, 1998), 10.

3. E. F. Nye, "Writing as Healing," *Qualitative Inquiry* 3 (1977): 1–9.

4. "She Reaches for Her Pen," *Prevention* 41 (1989): 1.

5. "How I Quit Stonewalling Step Four," *Lifeline Sampler* (1985) 82–83.

6. Ira Progoff, *At a Journal Workshop* (New York: Jeremy P. Tarcher, 1992).

7. S. W. Albert, *Writing from Life* (New York: Jeremy P. Tarcher, 1996), 9.

8. *Alcoholics Anonymous,* 4th ed. (New York: Alcoholics Anonymous World Services, 2001).

9. D. Danowksi and P. Lazaro, *Why Can't I Stop Eating?* (Center City, Minn.: Hazelden, 2000), 3.